Pranayama:

15 Step-by-Step Breathing Techniques to Relieve Stress and Calm Your Mind

Table of content:

Introduction: What is Pranayama?

Pranayama is a Sanskrit word, with "pran" meaning "breath", and "ayama" meaning "control". Breath control—sounds simple enough right? Just learning to control our breathing. But many of us have a much harder time with our respiration that we may realize. We rush from place to place, huffing and puffing, wheezing and panting. And as out of breath as we are, it often sends our entire body off-balance. You see, the quality of our breathing is much more important than we would care to admit.

Pranayama approaches the common practice of breathing as it were an artform, utilizing many centuries of respiratory perfection. For much of this time, the art of breathing—as it were—was mostly confined to monasteries in India, it wasn't until much more recently that this practice became known to the wider world. Pranayama was actually intensely guarded in mystical circles as a secret art, with most Yogi's (practitioners of Yoga) extremely reluctant to share their closely held secrets.

Usually, only the initiated who had proved themselves by passing several trials and tests were invited to learn more about pranayama. Previously it was only after a would-be adherent to pranayama subjected themselves to much fasting, and perhaps a few climbs of the Himalayan mountains with heavy rocks strapped to their backs, that these Yogic Masters shared their hidden knowledge. But you no longer have to climb Mt. Himalaya with a backpack full of rocks in order to train yourself in pranayama, the doors of knowledge have now been opened wide for anyone willing to venture in.

Chapter 1: Preparing for Pranayama

Before we begin our breathing exercises, there are a few things that you should prepare for in advance. You need to make sure that you are in the right place, and utilizing the right time, to make sure that your routine isn't interrupted, and that you get the most benefit from its practice. You also need to make sure that you are physically prepped with the right diet and sufficient rest so that you can be in the best condition to engage in a pranayama routine. Here in this chapter we will make sure that you learn the best way to prepare and optimize yourself for your pranayama breathing exercises.

Creating the Ideal Atmosphere for Pranayama

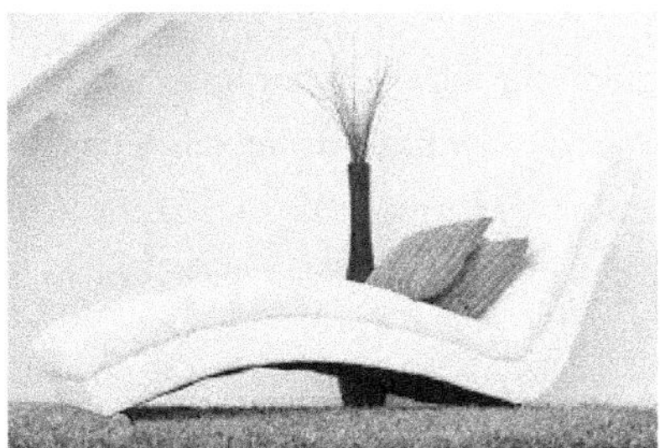

The Yogi's of old have spoken at great length when it comes to the ideal atmosphere in which pranayama should be practiced. Some of the recommendations that these ancient Indians crafted are largely irrelevant to us today, but other pieces of advice still hold true. Take this piece of ancient wisdom for example, the Yogi's always instructed followers of pranayama, that they should practice their breathing exercises, "in a province with a stable government, ruled by a kind, religiously minded ruler, stable government, ruled by a kind, religiously minded ruler and inhabited by religious masses."

For most in North America and Europe, such instructions are thankfully devoid of meaning, but in the ancient world where many regions were subject to invasion, ruthless dictatorships, and generally chaotic governments, such things had to be sorted out! Another piece of advice given about proper atmosphere is in much the same vein, stating, that there should be, "no fear of invasion and no disturbance from beasts, thieves, bad characters, insects, epidemics, and natural calamities like draught or floods."

This is again, a no brainer for most of us, and is basically stating, "Only do Pranayama in places where you won't get killed!" If you are planning on meditating in a back alley of the Bronx in New York, at 3 in the morning, its probably not a good idea. I think we can all understand that. But besides basic precautions for physical safety while engaging in Pranayama, what can we do? Number one, find a quite place. That means absolutely quiet, no TV, no radio, no conversations in the background.

You need to be in an environment where you can primarily focus on your breathing and not on other sounds reverberating around you. If your own living environment is unable to generate this kind of serenity, quiet corners of nature parks are a good place to practice, and so are private rooms in public libraries. But wherever you may go, just make sure that it is the ideal environment for pranayama.

Having Correct Posture and Seating

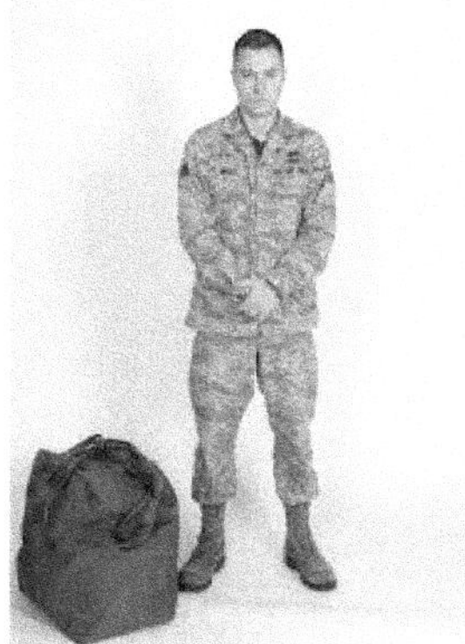

Next to creating the right atmosphere, the most important thing for any given breathing exercise is to have the right posture and seating while you perform it. You should make sure that the mind, as well as the joints, and muscles of the body are relaxed. If it helps you may want to engage in some brief stretching before you begin. Make sure you sit up straight, with your weight evenly balanced on your spine so that you can have the endurance to see your pranayama session through to the end.

Your body needs to be steady for prolonged meditative states, and pranayama is no different. If you are able, and it won't present any undue medical difficulties for you—you may also want to consider skipping breakfast as well. A full stomach tends to interrupt with the needed posture for pranayama. It is for this reason that it is often suggested to do pranayama early in the day before eating. Our lung capacity is also impacted by a full stomach, versus an empty one, so just keep all of these considerations in mind before you set out to do your breathing exercises.

Develop a Regular Pranayama Routine

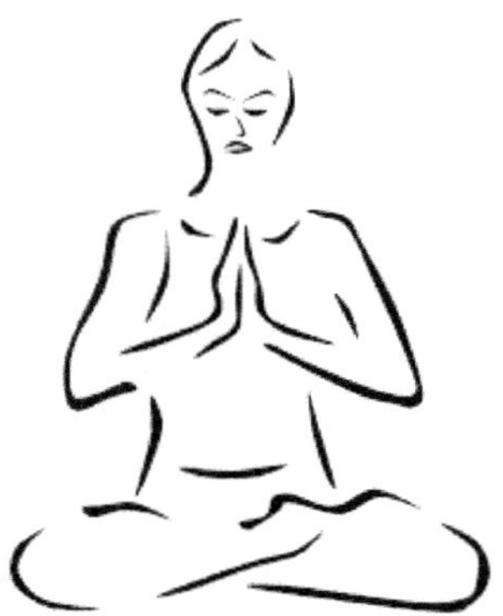

We all have routines. Even if it's just waking up in the morning, making a pot of coffee, and going into the shower, we all have set habits and routines that engage in during our life. One of the most important things that you can do in your preparation for pranayama is to simply prep for your own regular routine for your breathing exercises as well. Because the truth is, the benefits of pranayama will never be fully realized if you only do it on rare occasions.

You need to have regular times in which you can complete your exercises. This means setting aside a specific time either every day, or at least a few times a week, in which you can engage in the same repetitive exercises without interruption and without hindrance. Some really enjoy the fact that they can have designated times in which to focus on this aspect of their life. It enables them to get away for an hour a day without having to feel guilty. And if anyone asks any questions, just say— "Hey! Give me a break folks! It's just a part of my regular pranayama routine!"

Chapter 2: Practicing Abdominal and Diaphragm Breathing

Whether you actually practice the precepts of pranayama or not, it can't be stressed enough just how important abdominal breathing really is. The better we breathe out of our abdomen the better that we will generally feel. In pranayama, the breath that we breathe into ourselves is known as "Shwas", and the breath that we breath out is known as "Prashwas".

Using Pranayama Crocodile Breath

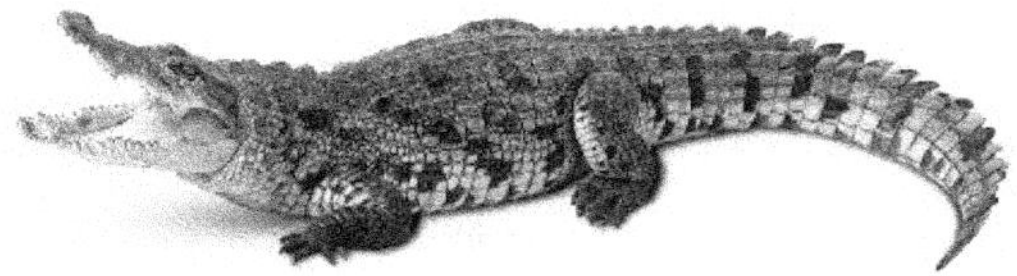

I know that some of you may be thinking that you have something akin to crocodile breath when you wake up in the morning but that is not what we are talking about here! When we refer to pranayama crocodile breath, we are actually referring to a very specific position that you can place upon the muscles of your diaphragm so that your breathing can be better facilitated. In order to place yourself into this position you need to lay flat on your stomach with your arms folded at about 45 degrees' high, over each shoulder. It may not be the most comfortable position at first, but your body will quickly acclimate to the unique stressors that this provides.

Once you are in this position you will feel your body's breath moving rapidly through your diaphragm and your abdomen. This breathing exercise will work to relieve abdominal tension that you may feel as you go throughout the day. Those that suffer from chronic anxiety typically have quite a bit of pressure in their abdomen when they breathe. Colloquially this is known as "butterfly's in the stomach". So, if you too could use a relief from those pesky butterfly's you should give pranayama crocodile breath a try! It will release the tension and set those butterfly's free!

Attaining the Relaxation Pose

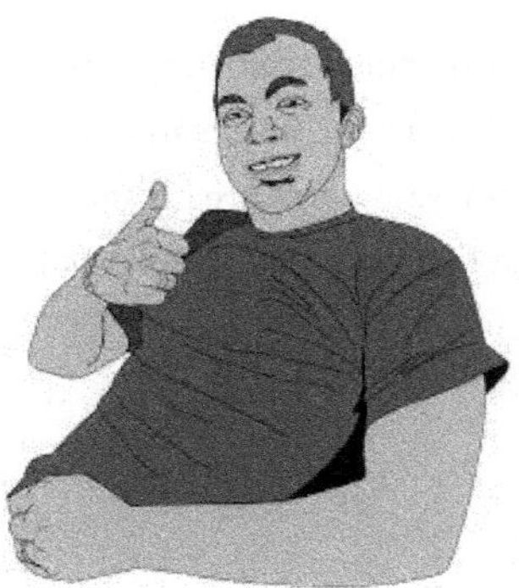

The relaxation pose, or as it is traditionally known in pranayama circles, "shavasana", is used to focus on abdominal breathing and particularly the abdomen as it rises and falls during relaxed and regular breaths. For this exercise, you will lay down, flat on your back, with your head slightly elevated by a pillow. Now begin to focus intensely on your breathing, making yourself acknowledge and experience every single movement as your lungs fill with air.

Let your rib cage become loose and flexible, even as the muscles of your body become still and devoid of all motion. After you have done this for a while, try raising your hands over your head as you breathe, serving as an extension of your rising abdomen as they rise and fall. Do this several times before putting your hands back down to your side. Now take a moment to continue breathing without this extra stimulation and monitor and take note of the changes in your respiration. You will immediately notice a feeling of great relaxation.

Upright Abdominal Breathing

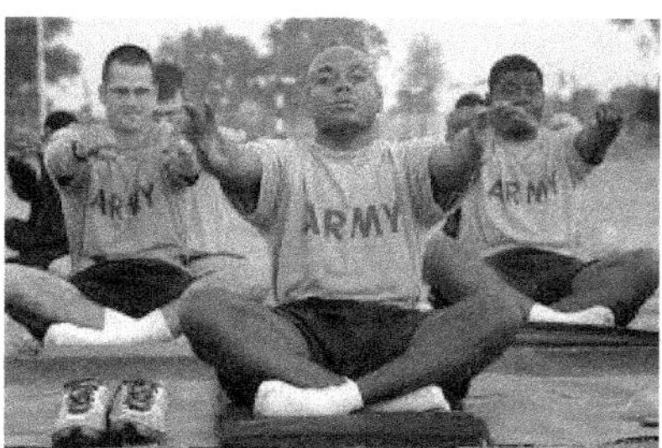

Just by sitting up in a chair you can experience a great change in your overall breathing capacity. From this change in position alone you will notice that your respiration does not feel like it does when you are standing, or lying in bed. This a clear indication of your diaphragm and abdomen at work, using muscles to help regulate breathing in a wide variety of physical poses. You can further enhance some of these techniques with regular breathing exercises. To engage in upright abdominal breathing, put each hand into onto your thighs as you are sitting upright in a chair.

Now close your eyes and pay especially attention to your abdomen and diaphragm as you breathe in and out. As you sit upright let your back muscles tighten slightly to keep your posture with minimum effort. You will soon notice your respiration expanding out on each side of your lungs. You will also see that your stomach is expanding with each and every breath. Proceed with this exercise for several more go arounds, carefully monitoring the sensations as you experience them. You should soon experience stronger more frequent breaths that seem to be coming from your upper abdomen. As you concentrate on your respiration allow your mind to relax.

Udara Svasana

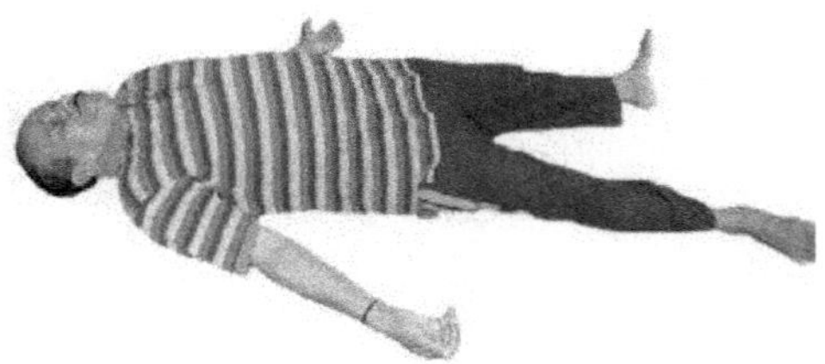

Udara Svasana is a traditional breathing technique that will allow the expansion of the abdomen. In this exercise, lay down flat on your back, stretched out on the floor. Next, place your hand over your belly button. Now inhale as deep as you possibly can, allowing your stomach to greatly expand from the air. As you do this, pay especial attention to your belly button. Watch as it lifts and recedes like the tides of the ocean, and you will soon see tidal waves of rest and relaxation flowing through you. All of the techniques presented in this chapter are greatly beneficial for redirecting respiration in the abdomen and diaphragm. Use them as much as they are needed.

Chapter 3: Pranayama Breathing

Pranayama breathing is a really unique way to improve physical and mental balance of the body. There are several techniques that can be explored to help facilitate relaxed respiration, but there are only so many pages in this book! Having that said, we are going to focus on the most important! Here in this chapter you will find the best of the best, try them all!

Bhastrika Pranayama

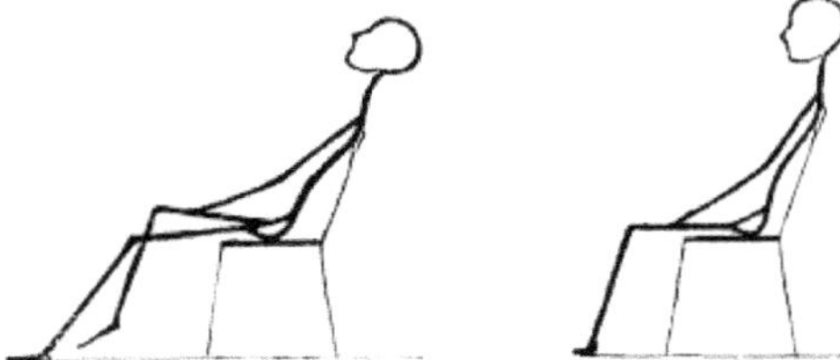

Also known as "bellows breath", "Bhastrika Pranayama" is a type of breathing exercise used to help increase your "prana" or as yoga gurus would have it—your life force. Such things are not to be taken lightly. Without adequate prana we become sluggish, slow, tried, and depressed. Sometimes we just need to recharge our prana batteries by improving our breathing. This exercise will allow you to do just that. Start off by placing yourself in a sitting posture on a hard-backed chair.

Raise yourself up as high as you can while maintaining good, straight posture in the seat. Now breathe in as deeply as possible, letting your abdomen fully expand as you do so. After doing this a few times, exhale with sudden force out of your nostrils, before inhaling just as forcefully. Repeat this several times. This will enable you to focus your respiration solely through your diaphragm, enabling you to send sudden surges of oxygen to your bloodstream, thereby giving you a sudden burst of energy.

I know that all this talk of "prana" and "life force" may sound like a bunch of mystical mumbo at first glance. But as you can see here, if we just change the terminology, much of what is practiced in exercises like this are very much based in very real, physiological science. This is precisely why—regardless of what your personal belief system might be—these yogic practices have some very real benefits for all of us, if we just give them a try for ourselves.

Kapalbhati Pranayama

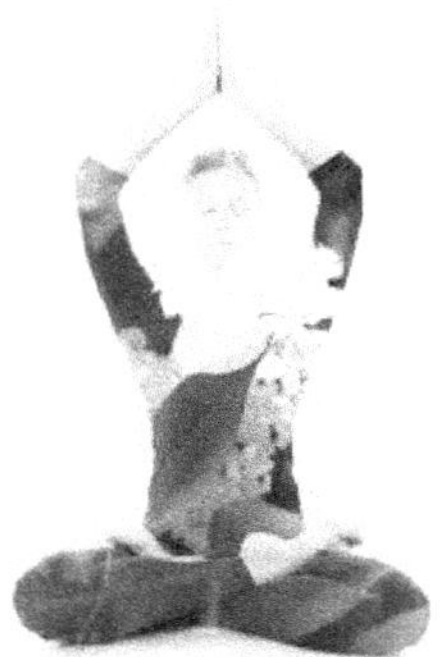

This yogic method of breathing will provide an immediate sense of calm and clarity to the mind. But rather than long breaths out of the abdomen, this method employs a series of focused, short and powerful exhalations, followed by a series of gentler inhalations. This method is meant to clean out the lungs, and there is quite a bit of evidence that this method really does help to filter out debris from mucous membranes in the respiratory system.

This method of breathing is especially helpful if you are suffering from allergies or cold and flu symptoms. This exercise has been said to bring about a "natural glow" in its participants, thus the explanation behind the yogic name for it, "skull shining breath". The best way to employ this exercise is to sit up straight, with your hands outstretched toward the ceiling, as you breathe in rapid breaths, followed by increasingly gentle, full inhalations.

Bahya Pranayama

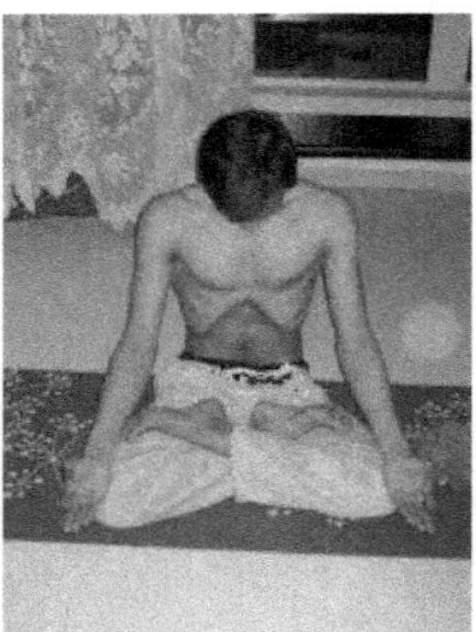

Also known as "external breathing" this method of pranayama, focusses on keeping our breathing outside of the body. How do you do that you might ask? Well—for starters make sure that you feel your diaphragm as it rises and falls, and your abdomen as it expands in and out. Keep a close focus on all of these aspects of your breathing throughout the entire experience. Now exhale with tremendous force, using your abdomen and diaphragm to squeeze as much air as possible outside of your lungs.

Next, touch your chin to your chest, and try to suck your abdomen in as much as you can (if you have ever been fat and tried to be skinny, you might know how to do this!) until your abdomen is perfectly retracted into your body. This exercise will leave you with a hollow space right below your ribcage, leaving your abdomen muscles firmly pressed against your back! Maintain this position as long as you can. Finally, lift your chin up and begin to slowly inhale, letting your lungs completely fill with air. Do this as many times as necessary.

Bramari Pranayama

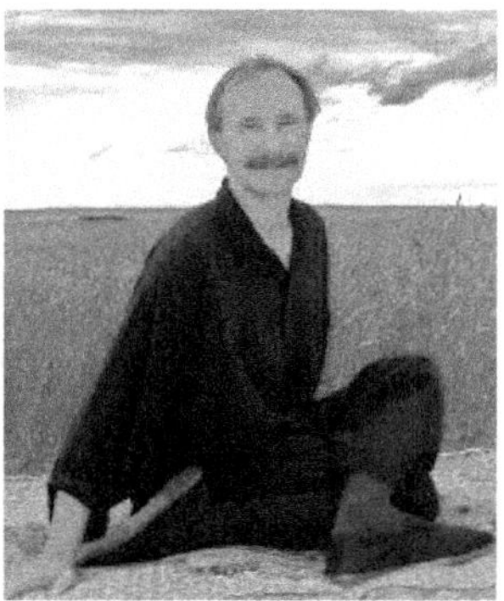

Bramari Pranayama is also sometimes known as "bee breath" and as you are about to see—for good reason. This type of exercise utilizes the vocal cords to create a loud intonation for the purpose of calm. The ancient yogic masters likened it to the bumbling of a bee. This breathing exercise provides great relief to any agitation or stress that you may be feeling. Try to sit as near as you can to a wall or corner, in order to help facilitate focus, and sit up straight in either a chair or right down on the floor.

Now place each one of your index fingers into your ear canals, and press down on the cartilage that resides between your ear and cheek. Inhale, and exhale; as you breathe out press down on this cartilage structure with your fingers. Do this while humming as loud as you can, sounding like something akin to a bee. Repeat this entire process several times until you feel better. On the surface this may seem like a really odd exercise, but it really does work! The only trouble is, when you are sitting at your cubicle in the middle of the day, holding your ears and buzzing like a bumble bee, your coworkers just might think you have lost your mind!

I can remember a time I was in the parking lot of a job I worked and became confronted with this sort of eventuality. I was behind schedule on a project and under severe duress and thought a little pranayama pick-me-up would help. As I looked out at the empty lot I thought I was by myself. I didn't see anyone walking around or in their cars, so I figured I had the all clear to do my thing. Well—everything was fine, until a security guard tapped on my window and asked, "Daughter just what do you think you are—a bumble bee?"

Needless to say, Mr. Security didn't quite have the patience for pranayama! But nevertheless, if you can manage it, without distraction or disruption, this one breathing exercise can do wonders to clear out stress! The actions involved in Bramari Pranayama serve to clear out frazzled nerves and bring back clarity and focus, you really should give this one a try!

<u>Purna Svasana Pranayama</u>

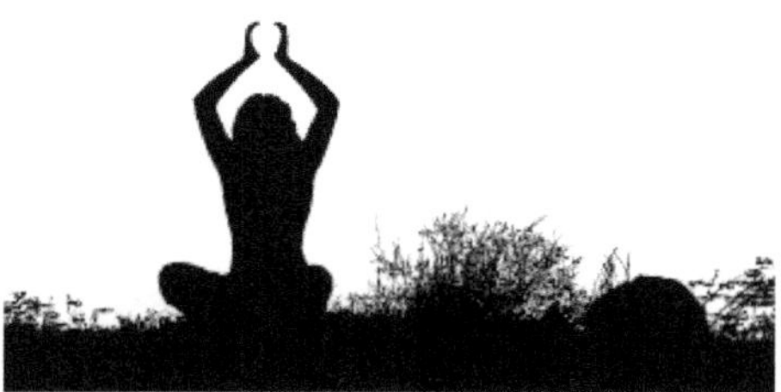

In order to engage in this breathing exercise seat yourself in a relaxed position, it doesn't' matter where, it could be on the floor or on the couch. Now lift each hand over your head and rest your arms on the back of each shoulder, with each elbow bended toward your head. This position will help to expand and stretch out your chest muscles to their maximum extent. Interestingly enough, those that are frequent sufferers of asthma have found this aspect of the exercise alone tremendously helpful in order to help free them from their often-constricted bronchial tubes.

As an asthma sufferer, I can personally vouch for this one myself. I often wake up unable to breathe, feeling like my lungs, or bronchial passages are closing up on me. Any asthma patient knows just how distressing this feeling is. With your bronchial tubes inside your lungs closing up into narrow little straws, no matter how much you struggle to breathe and get the air into your lungs, it remains stopped up in the back of your throat. Well there is indeed good news—because this exercise will help to open those gateways of air so that oxygen can better come in and out of the body.

<u>Cleansing Pranayama</u>

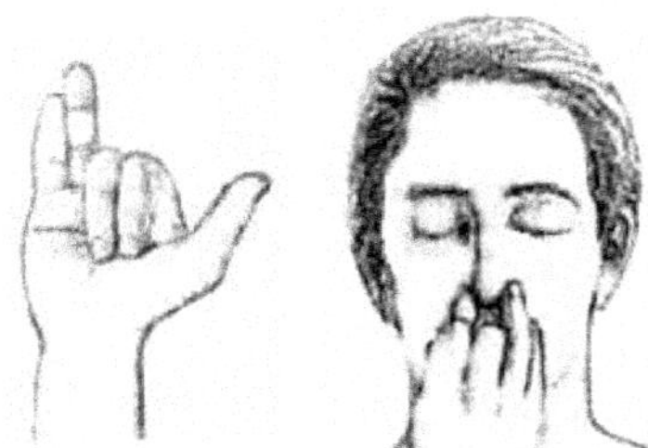

For this exercise you will need to sit in the standard "lotus" position with your legs crossed and your back completely straight. Now take your thumb and use it to close your right nostril, with your nostril closed in this manner, breathe in through your open left nostril. After you have done this, open your right nostril and close your left nostril. Now breathe out of your right nostril. Repeat this exercise several times before closing both nostrils and holding your breath for about 30 seconds or so.

As you continue to practice this routine attempt to expand that 30 second window of holding your breath for longer and longer periods of time. You can start off your first session with just 30 seconds, but then the next day, try 45 seconds, and the day after that a full minute. It is of course not recommended to hold your broth much longer than a minute. We are trying to reset and recalibrate the performance of our lungs after all—not trying to pass out! At any rate, if done correctly, this exercise will serve to help cleanse and calm your body's regulatory systems. It serves to improve the function of the nasal cavities in relation to the respiratory system.

Chapter 4: Tapping into the Head and Spine Circuits

In Pranayama, the head and spinal circuits refer to the centers of respiration that reside in the head, neck, and spinal column. These circuits should be utilized every single day in order to better facilitate proper pranayama breathing techniques. Here are a few of some of the most important circuits to make use of.

Spinal Breathing

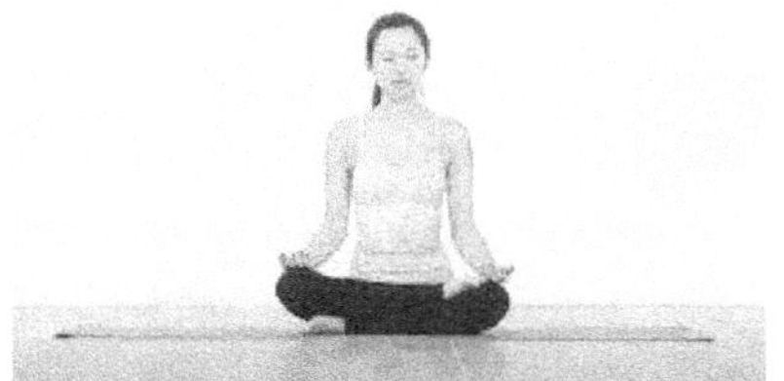

Sit in a comfortable position with each eye closed. Also keep your mouth shut as you inhale deeply though your nostrils. Make sure that inhalation begins through your abdomen and then proceeds to fill up your diaphragm, and then up your spine, across your collar bones and to your head. This form of spinal breathing allows the air to travel directly up your spinal circuit. This will improve your overall breathing capabilities tremendously. Be sure to make spinal breathing a part of your pranayama routine as soon as possible.

<u>Lion's Breath</u>

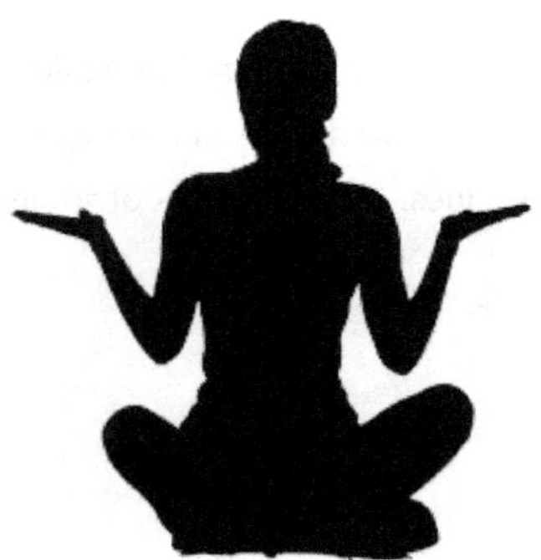

In this breathing exercise you can channel the ferocity of the lion in order to open up your breathing canal! Sit with your legs crossed on the floor and stretch out your hands with your palms upraised. Now look straight ahead with your eyes open wide, let your jaw slowly drop and then let out a lion's roar! Obviously, this technique requires a bit of privacy and can not be done where you will create a disturbance to others. But when you can find a good place to do it, lion's breath can really serve as a major relief to your respiratory system. After doing this exercise a few times you will notice that your throat is clearer, your eyes are more focused, and your general lung capacity has improved. All from a little lion's breath!

<u>*Dog Breathing*</u>

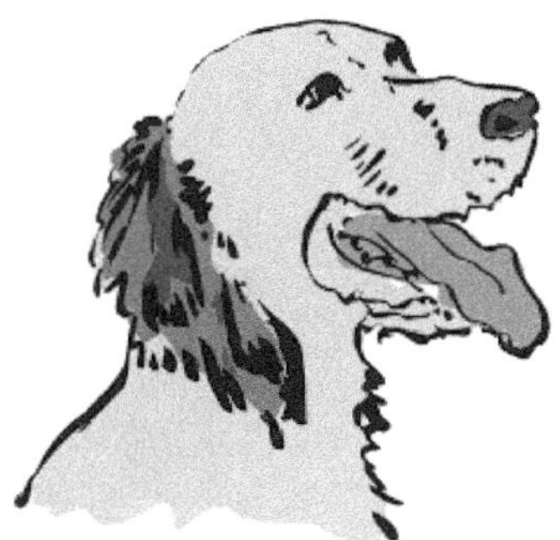

It may sound a little bit funny, but panting like a dog can have some tremendous benefits! Tapping into this head circuit will help you to catch your breath and increase your energy. And its just as simple as it sounds, when you have a nice and private place to practice, open your mouth, slightly distend your tongue and forcefully pant as you breathe in the air. In may not be the most attractive thing to do, but if you do it for long enough you will see some immediate results!

Applying Chin Lock

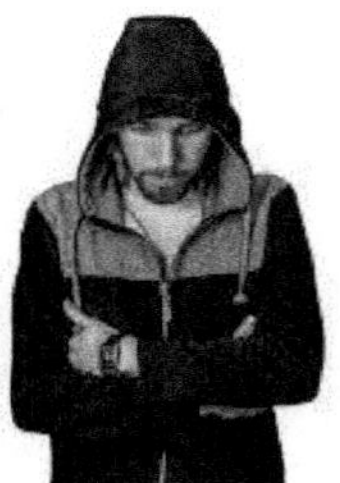

For those not exposed to pranayama, they may very well be wondering what a "chin lock" could be. In pranayama there are many ways that we can take advantage of special head and spine "circuits" or regions help facilitate our controlled breathing. And one of these ways to take advantage is to employ something called "chin lock". Using a chin lock entails putting the body in a state of relaxation, and after breathing deep and holding our breath, bending our head down so that our chin is firmly pressed, or "locked" into our chest.

After you have done this, now straighten out your hands right in front of you, press your knees together, and lock your position in place. Keep your breath held in, and maintain this pose for as long as you possibly are able to do so, in a relatively comfortable manner. Once you have held the position as long as you are able, you can then relax each shoulder, drop your arms, and raise your head out of the chin lock. Now allow yourself to exhale, breathing out slow and steady.

Rest for a moment and repeat. Harnessing this circuit will allow you to charge the neural pathways of your head and neck, pumping more blood to the region. It also helps to stimulate your thyroid glands, enabling them to better do their job of regulating the mood and stability of your mental state. This method has also been shown to help lower blood pressure for those who are suffering with higher from hypertension. Over all, practicing the chin lock will definitely be assistance to you, if you are battling against stress.

Rooting Yourself in Place

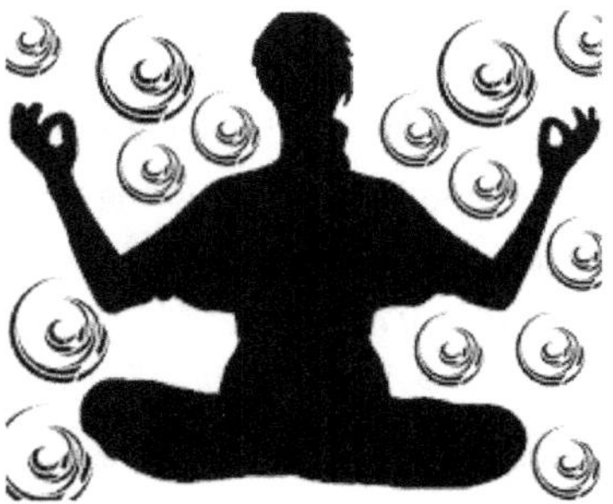

It is known as either "rooting your self in place" or simply the "root lock". This meditative pose is achieved with the knees reaching the ground, and the spine rigidly locked upright, and in place. Meanwhile the entire body is to begin a process of muscle relaxation with the palms outstretched before you. It is only then that the practice of pranayama can truly begin. No matter what kind of breathing technique you may be using, always make sure that you are firmly rooted in place before you begin—it is only then that the practice of pranayama can truly be carried out successfully.

Conclusion: Breathing Has Never Been Better!

If you don't mind me pointing out the obvious here, I just wanted to remind you of something—we all have to breathe. Breathing allows us to stimulate the life force within us, to keep us alive. Simply enough—if we didn't breathe we would not be able to continue living. But expand on that further, and you find that beyond just keeping our heart beating, the *quality of our breathing* in turn affects the *quality of our life.*

If we have constantly stressed and constricted lungs that force us to take short and shallow breaths, our mood and general health will almost certainly suffer as a result. The ancient yogis understood this connection and spent hundreds of years studying and perfecting something that most of us simply take for granted—how to breathe! They determined that "prana" was the underlying foundation behind all biophysical functions, and they sought to perfect it.

They knew from trial and error that through repetitive actions of the lungs, they could fortify and strengthen the entire body. With the routine practice of pranayama blood flow can be better regulated, the nervous system can be improved upon, and general health and vigor can be restored. And you too, can discover just as these ancient gurus found out thousands of years ago, just how beneficial a little bit of pranayama can be for you too! Thank you for reading!